TMJ No More

The Complete Guide to TMJ Causes,
Symptoms, & Treatments, Plus a
Holistic System to Relieve TMJ Pain
Naturally & Permanently

Jason S. Bradford
Copyright© 2014 by Jason S. Bradford

Publisher: Enlightened Publishing

ISBN-13: 978-1496080202

ISBN-10: 1496080203

Disclaimer

The Publisher has strived to be as accurate and complete as possible in the creation of this book. While all attempts have been made to verify information provided in this publication, the Publisher assumes no responsibility for errors, omissions, or contrary interpretation of the subject matter herein. Any perceived slights of specific persons, peoples, or organizations are unintentional.

This book is not intended for use as a source of legal, business, accounting or financial advice. All readers are advised to seek services of competent professionals in the legal, business, accounting, and finance fields.

The information in this book is not intended or implied to be a substitute for professional medical advice, diagnosis or treatment. All content contained in this book is for general information purposes only. Always consult your healthcare provider before carrying on any health program.

Table of Contents

Introduction: What is TMJ Disorder?

The temporomandibular joint is the joint that allows you to open and close the jaw. The joint connects the mandible or lower jaw to the upper jaw and face. This joint is known as the TMJ and is the only connection of the mandible to the rest of the body. The joint is a smooth "ball-in-socket" joint that is flexible enough to open and close the jaw, move the jaw from side to side and be able to accurately chew food. The muscles around the TMJ support the joint and control its movement and function.

The temporomandibular joint is located in front of your ears. When you open and close the jaw, you can feel the stretch of the skin overlying the joint. The joint normally has a smooth ball in joint movement. If you feel too much crunching and clicking of the joint, you might have TMJ syndrome.

The lower jaw or mandible consists of the "ball" part of the joint called the condyles. The socket is located on the temporal bone of the head, which is why the joint is called the temporo-mandibular joint. There is a soft disc between the condyle and the temporal bone that acts like a shock absorber to make the joint protected from certain movements and chewing behaviors.

The TMJ is one of the most complicated joints in the body because it has a hinge-type behavior and sliding mobility that makes it easy to malfunction. The jaw joint also has a complex system of muscles and ligaments that hold the joint together as it moves.

TMJ disorders can cause significant pain and dysfunction of the jaw joint. The muscles that control jaw movement can be too tight and this can cause stiffness of the joint. More than 20 million people in the US are believed to be affected by TMJ disorders. More women seem to have the problem when compared to men.

Most people have no pain or problems with the TMJ; however some will have cyclical pain in the joint that goes away without any treatment. Some people, on the other hand, will have long term symptoms associated with the joint and will become debilitated by the pain and inability to chew affectively.

TMJ syndrome is the result of stressors placed on the surrounding structures of the joint, including the disc cartilage, nearby ligaments, nerves, blood vessels, the muscles of the jaw, neck or face, and possibly the teeth. For many people who have TMJ disorders, there is no obvious cause or the cause is as yet unproven. Some unproven causes include having a poor bite, having problems with orthodontic braces, psychological stress, and grinding of the teeth.

People with poor posture can get TMJ syndrome. If you are one who sits forward all day staring at a computer screen or television, you can be at risk for TMJ disorder. Lack of sleep can play a role in the disease. If you have a muscular "trigger point" or tender spot located in the muscle of the facial area, this can cause you to have problems with your TMJ.

Arthritis of the TMJ, fractures of the face or mandible or frequent dislocation of the joint can trigger TMJ symptoms.

There are basically three types of pain associated with TMJ syndrome and they need to be approached differently from one another. These include:

- Internal derangement of the TMJ, such as a disc that has become displaced, an injury to the condyle or dislocation of the TMJ.
- Myofascial pain, which is pain to the muscles surrounding and controlling the joint (this is the most common source of TMJ pain).
- Arthritis in the joint itself, which can be degenerative in nature or inflammatory in nature.
- You can have any combination of these types of pain together, for example, inflammatory arthritis that is also associated with myofascial pain.

Many people have no particular cause for their TMJ syndrome, which makes treatment difficult. In fact, TMJ disorder is one of the most difficult facial diseases to treat. There are surgeries available for TMJ but these tend to cause more problems than they treat.

Interestingly, people with TMJ syndrome often have coexisting conditions including chronic fatigue syndrome, fibromyalgia or sleep problems. No one knows if these disorders have a common cause or exactly what the relationship is between these disorders and

TMJ disorder. Those with rheumatic diseases like rheumatoid arthritis can also get TMJ disorder as a secondary condition. Rheumatic diseases cause inflammation, pain and stiffness of the joints, bone and muscle. Both rheumatic conditions and TMJ issues can involve inflammation so they may be related in ways we don't know yet.

Because so little is known about TMJ disorders, allopathic doctors have little to offer those suffering from the disease. For this reason, many people suffer unnecessarily. This guide hopes to offer you ways to cope with temporomandibular joint disease so that the pain and debility of the disease is lessened. Many people suffer from TMJ disorder and there are probably many more who suffer without even telling their doctor.

There is hope for treating TMJ disorders so that you can eat normally, chew, bite down and be free of pain and abnormal sounds in your head. In this guide, we will talk about what you might be experiencing with TMJ disorder and which treatments, conventional or alternative, will control your pain, clicking sensation and stressful feelings.

***Melanie's Story:** I worked as a typist at a lawyer's office since I was 25 years old. I didn't realize that I was clenching my teeth when I typed and I think I had my desk set up wrong so it put extra pressure on my jaw. I began having pain in my head and I felt a clicking sensation in the joint in the front of my ear, which I later learned was my TMJ. Rather than seeking help from my family doctor, I sought the services of an alternative medicine doctor, who recommended kava for me as well as exercises. She showed me how not to clench my jaw when I was typing and told me how I could fix my workspace so my neck wasn't tilted wrong. I did everything she asked and got relief within a couple of weeks. I do my exercises faithfully and have no real pain.*

Chapter 1: TMJ Disorders Causes & Symptoms

Causes of Temporomandibular Joint Syndrome

No one knows the exact cause of TMJ disorder but it is suspected that many different causes are possible. Problems in the jaw muscles that protect the TMJ are believed to be the primary cause of the disease although arthritic changes can certainly cause some cases of the disease.

Bruxism or grinding of the teeth is a common problem that can lead to irritation and pain in the temporomandibular joint. Some people get bruxism only once in a while when they're stressed out over taxes or school. Others have it on a chronic basis and will not only have teeth damage but will have chronic headaches or pain in the TMJ area.

Those who have poor posture are at risk for TMJ disorder. If you hunch over a computer, you will damage your back and will push your jaw out of joint. This can lead to temporomandibular joint pain and crunching sounds coming from the TMJ. The lower jaw will shift forward, setting your teeth out of alignment and pushing your jaw joint (your TMJ) out of place. Pain and inflammation can set it so you have pain on opening and closing your jaw.

Teeth clenching from worrying and stress can contribute to extra stress on your temporomandibular joint. Stress itself seems to play a big role in getting the condition. The stress, of course, can be from anything and can take on many different forms, TMJ disorder being just one form.

You can have TMJ disorder from hyperextending your jaw, such as when you open your mouth too wide to eat a hamburger. Taking big bites can cause jaw muscle pain and can make TMJ disorder feel worse. If you have TMJ, you should keep your portions down to bite-sized quantities.

Interestingly, drug use can contribute to your getting TMJ disorder. If you use methamphetamines or cocaine, you're prone to getting teeth clenching symptoms and teeth grinding. This alone can cause TMJ symptoms or can make TMJ symptoms worse.

Injury to the jaw or the muscles of the jaw can result in TMJ disorder. Blows happen in car accidents—or whiplash—which can trigger you to have jaw pain that leads to TMJ syndrome.

You can dislocate the soft, cushioning disc in the joint itself. This allows bone to rub against bone and increased pain in the joint affected by the dislocation. Sometimes this can be repaired surgically but it doesn't always work.

Osteoarthritis or bone spurs can cause worsening pain in the area of the TMJ so that bone rubs on bone and you experience grinding or crackling sensations in your TMJ, which can secondarily become inflamed and increase in pain.

It's important to note that in most cases, the doctors never find out what the cause is of the TMJ syndrome. It's possible that a variety of causes converge together to cause the disease and that there just isn't one cause affecting the joint.

The bite itself is a big part of getting TMJ syndrome. When the teeth are not in alignment, it pulls the muscles out of place and the joint becomes damaged because it doesn't line up correctly. Just getting older and having teeth go out of alignment can play a role in getting the disease. Using the teeth for things for which they are not intended—called parafunction—can cause the teeth to have uneven chewing surfaces and a TMJ joint that does not line up correctly.

Autoimmune diseases can play a role in getting TMJ syndrome. These types of diseases lead to low grade inflammation in just about every joint in the body. Overusing the TMJ joint in any way can subsequently trigger pain and inflammation of the joint.

Symptoms of Temporomandibular Joint Syndrome

TMJ can be mild, moderate or severe. It can be a temporary pain, an intermittent pain, or a steady pain that can last for many years. It is experienced more in women but no one knows why this is the case. The age at onset is somewhere between the ages of 20 and 40.

Common symptoms include:

- Pain or tenderness of the facial area, especially near the joints, neck, shoulders or around the ear area.
- A "locked" or "stuck jaw, especially when it is stuck in the open position. It can also be locked in the closed position but not with the right bite.
- Inability to open the mouth very wide can be from TMJ disorder.
- Clicking sensations, popping sensations or grating sensations are common with TMJ disorder, especially when opening and closing the mouth.
- Feeling "tired" in the facial area.
- A suddenly uncomfortable bite—as though the teeth aren't fitting quite together.
- Swelling just in front of the ear in the upper outer cheek region
- Toothaches in the upper teeth
- Headaches or migraines that are unresponsive to rest and pain medications
- Ringing sensation in the ear—a condition called tinnitus
- Dizziness
- Earaches
- Upper shoulder pain

Of all of the above complaints, pain in the muscles responsible for chewing is the most major. People who have the condition often complain of a dull aching sensation in the face, particularly near the TMJ area although referred pain is also possible to the ears, shoulders, forehead and neck. The pain tends to be more noticeable in the morning hours or in the late afternoon hours. The teeth can be sensitive in the absence of any real dental pathology or you can have an earache with no ear infection or redness.

It's not uncommon for patients who suffer from TMJ syndrome to see many different specialists in a quest for understanding of what's happening including ear specialists, throat specialists, neurologists, chiropractors and pain specialists. Often, it is the simple dentist or primary care specialist who puts it all together and identifies the problem as simply TMJ syndrome.

Diagnosis of TMJ

There is no true diagnostic protocol for temporomandibular joint syndrome and no widely acceptable standardized test for the disease. For the most part, the doctor looks at the symptoms and the physical examination, careful to rule out any other possible cause of the pain, such as tooth decay or migraine headaches. Other possible sources of the pain include sinus infections and ear infections.

The doctor or dentist will perform a "clench test" in which you bite down or clench your teeth to see where the pain is. If some or all of your teeth are in pain, then you need to consider the possibility of a bad bite or a tooth cause of TMJ syndrome.

X-rays of the teeth and TMJ can be taken which may show a bad bite or arthritic changes/dislocation of the TMJ. Molds can be taken of the teeth to demonstrate the bite of the teeth. In addition, there is a computerized bite analysis test known as a T-Scan that will tell if there are dentition or bite problems. A CT or MRI scan of the head can show abnormalities of the temporomandibular joint. The MRI can check to see if the TMJ disc is in proper alignment.

The doctor or dentist may check the TMJ for clicking or popping sounds and might do a panoramic x-ray to see if the TMJ is sound or not. If all other conditions have been ruled out, then TMJ syndrome is the most likely diagnosis.

Mark's Story: *I first knew I had TMJ syndrome when I tried to bite into a large hamburger and my jaw locked shut. It was so painful and I couldn't get it unlodged. I went to the emergency room and they unlocked the jaw. I continued to have pain, particularly on the right. I went to my doctor and got referred to have an MRI exam. The doctor told me I had a dislocated meniscus, which is the spongy cushion that makes the TMJ move more smoothly. In the end, I had to see a surgeon who did arthroscopic surgery on me. He fixed my meniscus and, while I still had a little pain on occasion after that, I am much better and now no longer eat such big sandwiches.*

Chapter 2: Conventional Treatments

Because it is difficult to determine the actual cause of TMJ disorder, it is hard to find a conventional cure that works for everyone. There is a lot of hit and miss when it comes to treating this disorder.

There are some simple and conservative measures you can take for TMJ disorder. These include applying moist heat to the joints themselves or applying cold packs. Some people alternate hot and cold packs every half hour. Other practitioners recommend only ten minutes of ice to the TMJ at a time.

There are simple and relaxing stretching exercises that can be taught to you by a physical therapist, doctor, or dentist. Exercise your jaw twice to three times a day and then put a warm, moist washcloth or towel on the TMJ on either or both sides. Hold the cloth on your affected joints for 5-10 minutes. It will soothe the joint and temporarily ease your pain.

Try to eat soft foods like mashed potatoes, yogurt, soup, scrambled eggs, fish, cottage cheese, beans, grains and vegetables that have been cooked thoroughly. Make sure your food is cut into small pieces so you don't need to open and close your mouth too wide. Don't eat crunchy or hard foods like raw carrots, peanuts, pretzels and hard rolls. Avoid chewy foods like taffy and caramels and avoid large foods that require you to open your mouth really wide.

The mainstay of medications for temporo-mandibular joint disease are medications like Tylenol, which relieves pain and nonsteroidal anti-inflammatory medications (NSAIDs) that work for pain and inflammation. These include Advil®, Motrin® and Aleve® (naproxen). They can be taken several times a day as directed for pain relief.

Muscle relaxants can be used for people who clench their teeth too much. It helps relax tight jaw muscles so that there isn't so much pressure on the joint and the bite isn't too tightly misplaced. Some people take anti-anxiety medications because it relaxes them and therefore, their joints. Anti-anxiety agents also help relieve stress, which is believed to play a role in getting TMJ disorder. Low dose tricyclic antidepressants have a strong track record for controlling chronic pain and are often used in patients with this kind of pain. Other than the pain medications that are available over the counter, the rest need a doctor's prescription.

Low level laser therapy can be used to treat pain and inflammation of various body areas, including the TMJ area, by providing local heat to the area. It can also be used to increase your neck's range of motion and your ability to open your mouth easily.

There are splints or night guards you can use. They involve plastic molded items that fit over the upper and lower jaw to prevent clenching of the teeth or grinding of the teeth. Such splints can correct the bite so that the teeth are not traumatized. Splints are usually worn all the time, while night guards are used only when you sleep. You usually work with a dentist to get a well-formed splint or night guard to use when you need it.

Corrective treatments by a dentist can be used to make sure your biting surfaces fit right. For example, you may need to have crowns, braces or bridges to make sure you have a perfect bite that doesn't interfere with your TMJ.

Doctors recommend that you avoid extreme movements of the jaw, such as chewing gum, yawning or chewing of ice. Even things like yelling and singing can aggravate the temporomandibular joint and surrounding musculature. Don't even rest your chin on your hand or hold the phone between the shoulder and the ear. This can overstretch the muscles and ligaments associated with the TMJ.

Try to keep your teeth slightly apart from the upper and lower jaw. This practice will eliminate the pressure on the joints and will eliminate bruxism.

There are some higher tech ways to treat TMJ syndrome. These include using a TENS unit, also called transcutaneous electrical nerve stimulation. This involves electrodes that are placed over the TMJ on the affected sides that are attached to a unit that sends low grade electrical signals to the electrodes. The electrical signals override the pain signals and you experience less pain. It actually works quite well for some individuals but it is not something you want to be seen out in public wearing.

Deep heating ultrasound treatments can be applied to the TMJ. After the treatment, you have reduced tenderness and pain. You will also temporarily have an increase in mobility of the TMJ.

Injection Relief for TMJ

Some doctors recommend trigger point injections. This involves the injection of various agents (to be discussed) into the TMJ itself or surrounding areas. Some of these treatments are considered off-label and are not actually recommended by the US Food and Drug Administration (FDA) so you need to talk to your doctor about the purpose of the injection and the safety of injecting the chosen medication into your TMJ area before going ahead with getting the injection.

Botox or Botulinum toxin type A is a drug made from the Botulinum toxin—a toxin produced by the same bacteria that causes food poisoning. It has been used for specific eye disorders like blepharospasm, neck spasms, and serious underarm sweating. While not approved for use in TMJ disorder, it can be injected into the muscles surrounding the

TMJ, relaxing the muscles and taking the tension off the TMJ. Doctors don't know exactly how it works but suspect that, by relaxing the muscles, you can take away some of the forces that are causing the TMJ to be too tight.

For inflammation relief, there are steroid injections or injections of hydrocortisone preparations. These act directly on the joint itself in order to ease inflammation of the joint. This is especially true if the joint is being affected by rheumatoid arthritis or even degenerative joint disease. Some preparations of cortisone last up to three months with inflammation and pain relief. It cannot however be used more than three times per year and it is still considered a controversial treatment.

A hyaluronan or hyaluronic acid injection can be used to treat osteoarthritis of the TMJ joint. It has its greatest usefulness for the management of knee or hip arthritis, but is used off label for those who have severe arthritis of the TMJ. It is still relatively controversial when it is used to treat arthritic temporomandibular joints.

Local anesthetic drugs can be used to inject into the TMJ. Some local anesthetics are more long acting than others and will relieve pain for a few days. Sometimes a local anesthetic can be used for the diagnosis of exactly where the pain originates from so it can be used for other types of treatment. The FDA has not approved local anesthetics as agents to inject into the TMJ.

Ozone therapy involves an ozone gas injection into the temporomandibular joint. The idea is that ozone can reduce inflammation and stimulate cartilage growth in the joint. In addition, it can kill pathogens like bacteria, fungi and viruses that contribute to bodily inflammation. This is a therapy that is also not approved by the FDA.

Sclerotherapy is another non-approved therapy for TMJ. It involves taking an irritant solution and injecting it into a muscle tendon or ligament near the TMJ. The sclerosing agent induces the proliferation of brand new cells so that the weakened ligaments are made stronger. Stronger ligaments improve the pain in the TMJ. The problem with this therapy is that not all TMJ problems are the result of weakened ligaments and it isn't clear whether strengthening weak ligaments do anything at all to alleviate the pain of this disorder. This is a treatment that is not FDA-approved. This type of therapy is also called prolotherapy.

Radio wave therapy involves sending a low level of electrical stimulation directed at the joint. This increases blood flow to the joint, so the patient will have a decreased sensation of pain. It can be used on one or both TMJs at the same time.

Surgical Relief for TMJ

Surgical relief for TMJ is generally reserved as a last resort treatment. It is used by doctors whenever all other therapies have been proven to be non-efficacious. Before getting surgery, seek a second or third opinion as to whether this will help your symptoms of pain and clicking sensation in the TMJ area.

There are three major types of surgery, including arthrocentesis, arthroscopy and open-joint surgery. The surgery you get usually depends on the type of problem you are having.

In an arthrocentesis, general anesthesia is necessary. It is reserved for instances where the person has a sudden onset of closed locked joint so the mouth will not open. Patients with this problem generally have not had a prior history of TMJ issues. Needles are inserted into the TMJ joints and the joint is washed out with sterile liquids. A blunt tool is sometimes swept across the joint on the inside so that anything that is creating an adhesion band within the joint can be dislodged. If a disc is dislodged in a certain way, the blunt instrument can move it to its proper position.

In an arthroscopy, a small device with a camera is inserted into the joint using general anesthesia. The lighted camera is hooked up to a video screen so that everyone in the surgical suite can see what's going on in the joint. Inflamed tissue and the disc and condyle can be removed or repaired using instruments attached to the arthroscope. This is considered to be a less invasive procedure than an open surgery and just about the same things will be able to be done with an arthroscope as with open surgery. The recovery time is short and there is minimal bleeding. The one downside is that it takes a skilled surgeon to be able to do this procedure and it might not be successful in relieving your pain.

Sometimes the problem is too severe and open joint surgery is necessary. This also done under general anesthesia. The entire area surrounding the TMJ is opened up and several different things can be done to the TMJ area. It is a procedure that is necessary if the bony aspects of the TMJ are deteriorating, if there happens to be tumors in the area of the TMJ, or if there is severe scarring or bone chips within the joint itself. There is a much longer healing time when compared to arthroscopy and a greater incidence of nerve damage and scar tissue.

It is possible to replace the entire temporomandibular joint with an artificial joint— condyle or ball-side of the joint. This is something you want to do after a great deal of consideration because it is a big surgery with a long recovery time and a chance that you will just trade one kind of TMJ pain for another. There are different TMJ implantation devices your doctor might choose from and you need to research the type of device you are getting, including reviews on how it has worked for others in the past. You need to know that many people still have pain after TMJ replacement surgery but that it is a different type of pain than the pain you had with TMJ syndrome. Talk to your doctor and get second opinions before going so far as to have a TMJ replacement surgery.

Conventional therapy is possible with TMJ but it is woefully ill-prepared to do so without potential harm to the delicate structure of the joint. Seek the advice of a craniofacial surgeon, a facial plastics surgeon or a dentist who specializes in TMJ before making a decision to have injections or complicated surgical therapy to correct your TMJ pain. Don't forget trying the common remedies first.

Amy's story: I was first diagnosed with bruxism when I was 21. This is a condition where you grind your teeth unconsciously, often in your sleep. It must have thrown off my bite and caused increased tension in the jaw. I started having increased pain and stiffness in the TMJ on both sides. It got so bad that I couldn't open my mouth for larger foods and I had to eat soft foods like cottage cheese and yogurt. That's when I saw a maxillofacial surgeon. He recommended Botox injections into the muscles around the TMJ. The result was relaxation of the muscles and the ability to eat foods I hadn't been able to eat for a long time. Then I was fitted with a splint I could wear that prevented the bruxism. I wore the splint and the muscles never tensed up again. I was happy I didn't have to have invasive surgery for my TMJ problem.

Chapter 3: Alternative Treatments

Given the fact that conventional medicine has few answers as to the cause and treatment of TMJ syndrome, many people are turning to alternative treatments to take care of their painful condition. There are many different alternative medical treatments that can aid the condition and cure the pain.

Some of these include:

Acupuncture

This is an ancient Chinese technique for healing that is based on balancing the life energy in the body—an energy called "Qi" or "chi". When chi is balanced, certain areas of the body have chi flow through them better and pain or discomfort is relieved.

The skin is prepared with alcohol and very thin, solid needles are inserted into specific areas of the skin, sometimes near the site of the TMJ and sometimes distant from the site of the TMJ. The needles are twirled with the hands or have electrical stimulation applied to it so that the channels of chi can be opened. It often takes several rounds of acupuncture in order to affect some kind of relief of pain. It can genuinely work for you if you use a well-trained acupuncturist.

Biofeedback

Biofeedback is often used when pain is at issue or when stress is a problem. With biofeedback, body responses such as skin temperature, blood pressure, muscle tension or heart rate can be altered just through the power of the mind. You need to practice biofeedback by using monitors such as skin sensors or muscle tension sensors so that you can find the right state of mind to affect these bodily functions.

Biofeedback allows you to calm your muscles and your mind so you feel less stress and feel less pain in your TMJ because the muscles have been trained to relax. You initially do this in a clinic or laboratory so the sensors can guide your ability to control whatever body function you're interested in, such as your muscle tension in the face. You can then learn to train your brain to act in the same way in the future. Your muscles will be relieved of tension automatically.

Chelation Therapy

Chelation therapy is a unique treatment based on the belief that many disorders, including TMJ disorder, arterial disease, high blood pressure, depression and fibromyalgia are partially caused by an elevated level of toxic heavy metals in the system. Some of these heavy metals include lead (in older homes), mercury (in dental fillings), thallium and cadmium. Exposure to these kinds of heavy metals has been known to be toxic to humans and animals.

In chelation therapy, IVs are used to give the affected patient benign binding agents. The binding agents will bind heavy metals in the bloodstream and tissues, and the combination of heavy metal and binding agent are flushed through the kidneys.

Chiropractic

Chiropractic services are generally used to treat neck, midback and lower back spine disorders but can be used to treat all areas of the musculoskeletal system. It is based on the idea that subluxations of the neck, which are minor neck dislocations, will cause TMJ disorder. The neck is made better through manipulation.

In addition, the chiropractor can do manipulation of the TMJ itself and can release muscle spasms that can cause the tension of the joint. They can practice electrical stimulation therapy or heat therapy to the joint that can relieve the pain.

Craniosacral Therapy

This is a type of manual therapy that involves slight movements to the cranial or head bones. Because the mandible and temporal bone are both "head" bones, they can be affected by craniosacral area, although other bones can be affected at the same time.

The therapist places their hands on the patient in order to tune into the person's craniosacral rhythm and adjusts the bones. This form of therapy has been used to treat TMJ syndrome, migraine headaches, fibromyalgia, stress and pain in the neck, midback, and lower back. The nervous system is said to be in better "harmony" after craniosacral therapy.

Homeopathy

There are several homeopathic remedies used for the treatment of TMJ syndrome. Homeopathy is a form of therapy that gives extremely small doses of a chemical that would otherwise make the person sick if given in higher doses.

In order to have relief with homeopathy, you need to see a homeopathic doctor who will examine you and decide on a remedy to dilute into small quantities and then give you a bottle of low dose medication to take. It often takes a few days or weeks to have any relief from this type of therapy but some people have found relief from homeopathy.

Naturopathy

This is a practice of medicine based on the belief that the body has an innate capacity to heal from injury or illness. It is based on believing in vitalism, which means that there is vital energy inside everyone that takes care of all bodily functions, including metabolism, adaptation and growth. A holistic approach is used and there is a strong belief in noninvasive treatment of disease.

There are both traditional naturopathic doctors and naturopathic physicians that work within the confines of conventional medicine but use it in a natural way. The practice has been alive since the 1890s but became more popular since the 1970s. Various modalities are used in naturopathic medicine, some of which are not accepted by conventional medicine.

Yoga

Yoga is an ancient Asian form of exercise that works extremely well for people with stress-related diseases. TMJ disorder can be relieved by the practice of yoga. This form of exercise involves the performance of "asanas" or poses that relax the mind and body.

The asanas are done along with special breathing techniques designed to make the asanas more relaxing. The most common type of yoga used in the US is Hatha yoga, which involves measured breathing and mostly static poses designed to refresh and relax a person. Pain can actually be relieved by being better rested and less stressed.

Meditation

Meditation is an alternative way to relax and relief stress and pressure off your mind. You basically find a focus for your mind such as a word or an image and allow your breathing to relax you, thinking pleasant and peaceful thoughts.

Meditation can be used specifically for pain management and is used by alternative and conventional medicine modalities alike. It is sometimes used along with yoga or is practiced by those who also practice yoga with great success in relieving stressful causes of pain.

It's important to remember that much of TMJ syndrome comes from the clenching or grinding of teeth and that those alternative or conventional medical therapies that reduce stress will reduce the incidence of teeth clenching or grinding. This, in turn, relieves the pain and inflammation of TMJ disorder. Things like progressive muscle relaxation, deep breathing exercises, self-hypnosis and guided imagery help to reduce stress. You not only feel better about yourself but your pain is improved as well. Any pain you do have left over is handled much better when you are in charge of your body through stress-reducing techniques.

If you can't do stress-relieving techniques on your own, try joining a class that teaches meditation, yoga, guided imagery or other stress-reducing measures. See an alternative medicine specialist for advice and treatment if you wish to use some of their techniques. The ultimate goal is pain reduction and self-sufficiency when it comes to your TMJ symptoms.

Some people with TMJ disorder use what's called the *Alexander Technique* for pain and stress reduction. This is a technique developed in the 1890s by Frederick Alexander. He used the technique to get rid of hoarseness as he was a public speaker. The technique makes use of postural habit changes that can affect the muscles of the head and neck especially. It reduces chronic stiffness in various muscles by learning how to mindfully move through life. It shakes off many people's inefficient ways of moving and patterns of tension so that you are more relaxed, relieving facial pain. The treatment is not completely passive and you have to go through the program or read a book about it to learn the skills set that it takes to help you feel freer and more grounded in life.

The Alexander Technique involves improving the ways you move, balance yourself, support yourself and have coordination. It helps you use just the right amount of energy for most of your activities so that you have energy left over for everything you need to do in your life. It releases unnecessary tension, whether you are sitting, standing, lying down, lifting or doing some other activity.

Any time you are attempting to rid yourself of TMJ pain using alternative methods, you should contact your regular allopathic doctor to make sure that nothing about the alternative therapy will interfere with treatment you are already taking. Make sure you remain wary of anything that says it will "cure your problems" as TMJ disorder is a chronic illness that is managed over a period of time. Because TMJ disorder is a complex disease, a multidisciplinary approach with both allopathic treatments and alternative treatments is recommended.

Samantha's Story: *I was diagnosed with TMJ disorder when I started developing pain in my jaw and had almost daily headaches. My doctor diagnosed me with the disease after I had had symptoms for more than 6 months. He also was the kind of doctor who did acupuncture and he recommended it for my TMJ pain and headaches. He said the two were related. I went through six acupuncture treatments total and felt resolution of my pain. My doctor also recommended yoga so I could learn to relax my body, including my jaw muscles. I took up yoga while I was still taking acupuncture treatments. When the treatments stopped, the yoga exercises took over and helped me learn poses that relaxed my face and kept the pain of TMJ disorder from coming back. I still do yoga and have had no reoccurrence of my pain.*

Chapter 4: TMJ Relief with Nutrition & Diet

Most people don't think of nutrition or diet when thinking of TMJ but it can make all the difference between suffering with the disease and learning how to live with it. Stress is considered to be one of the main causes of TMJ along with a bad bite. The question is: how do we use nutrition and dietary changes to affect change in the symptoms of TMJ disorder?

This chapter will delve into nutrition and TMJ disorder, including providing you with some tasty recipes that are known to help you learn to cope with this frustrating disease. The recipes work because they don't require you to bite down hard and will not worsen the disease.

When stress is a factor in your getting TMJ, a breakfast of protein is an excellent idea. It increases your emotional resistance, makes you feel full and provides your mental and physical "gas tank" with the fuel it needs to start the day. Protein sources for breakfast include sausage patties, eggs, fish and cheese. Protein drinks are also acceptable or you can use whey powder in fruit juice or blended into a smoothie with yogurt and fruit. Refined sugar and caffeine can cause you to clench your teeth too much, which will make you have greater TMJ symptoms.

There are nutritional supplements you can take that help TMJ that is stress-related. These include:

- Vitamin B Complex –This is a great stress buster for TMJ relief.
- Multi-mineral chelates or citrates—These help buffer acids that accumulate during stress. They also relax your muscles.
- Co-enzyme Q10—This provides you with healing energy.
- Omega 3 Fatty Acids—These have anti-inflammatory properties.
- Glucosamine sulfate—This is for good joint health.
- Vitamin C in doses of 2000 mg/day—This is anti-inflammatory for joint

health and will rebuild connective tissue near your joints.

Many people with TMJ disorder have fought their disease on their own, looking for and finding things that seem to help the symptoms. One such choice for TMJ is called "Anti-TMJ Broth". It works because it contains hyaluronic acid which can help improve joint function. The recipe for the soup is listed below:

Anti-TMJ Broth

This soup is made from the knuckle bones of cattle or from chicken breasts. It stimulates digestion and improves the intake of other nutrients you take in. The connective tissue contains hyaluronic acid that improves TMJ joint function. You can make this soup using a Crockpot, stovetop or microwave. The soup can contain any or all of the following:

- Meat as described above
- Okra
- Squash pieces
- Greens of some kind
- Celery

- Asparagus
- Canned beans of any kind
- Red peppers or green peppers

Season with salt and pepper or with some tomato paste. Simmer all ingredients together and remove any bony parts of the soup before eating. It is a healthy soup useful for all year round. Eat a bowl of soup for lunch and for dinner for the best results.

Other recommendations for TMJ sufferers?

Cut back on wheat and dairy products, including whole grain foods. Eat fewer foods with sugar, yeast and lots of preservatives. Use fewer salicylates, which block vitamin K activity. Eat red meat (well pulverized) that contains vitamin B12, iron, and zinc. Organ meat is sometimes good to eat as it contains micronutrients. Vegetable stew with soft vegetables and cooked beans are easy to eat and not hard on the TMJ.

The gist of eating with TMJ disorder is to eat foods that are soft to eat, not crunchy and not chewy. There are foods that work well for bruxism, which is the grinding of the teeth that can contribute to TMJ disorder. Supplements have their place in that many are anti-inflammatory, antioxidant and relax the body's muscles.

Other nutritional supplements that haven't so far been mentioned include MSM, SAMe, L-tyrosine, hops, feverfew, skullcap and passion flower. Hops, for example, is an excellent calmative and relaxant known to get rid of insomnia, nervousness and other stress-related symptoms. Talk to a reputable herbalist about this and other herbs that can help TMJ syndrome.

Some people with TMJ disorder get better with a hypoglycemic diet or one that his high in fiber and protein but that is low in plain sugar. There are plenty of fresh vegetables and fruits in this diet as well as legumes and starchy vegetables. Starchy vegetables and sweet fruits should be eaten in moderation.

The low sugar diet cuts down on grinding of the teeth because you aren't revved up so much on sugar. Eat small meals several times a day instead of big meals and keep your bites small. Avoid products high in caffeine including coffee and tea; avoid alcoholic beverages. Try to have low levels of sugar in your system by the time you go to bed so you don't grind your teeth in your sleep. Remember that high fructose corn syrup contains sugar and will have the same effect that sugar has.

There is a theory that was proposed more than 70 years ago by Weston A. Price that says that giving a child a great deal of sugar during development causes the child to develop deformed dental arches. This, in turn, causes the child to develop TMJ disorder later in life. There is no way to fix the problem if you had high sugar levels as a child but you can protect your children from eating too much sugar.

Many who suffer from bruxism and TMJ disorder seem to have low levels of the B vitamins. You should consider a multivitamin that contains at least 200 milligrams of each of the major B vitamins per day. This should reverse any deficiency and may also help improve symptoms of TMJ disorder.

Recipes for TMJ Disorder Patients

Let's look at some recipes that are intended to help those with TMJ disorder eat well, get the nutrients they need and won't cause bruxism or chewing too hard.

Tender Delicious Ribs

Ingredients:

- 2 racks of baby back ribs, pork or beef
- 1 cup barbecue sauce
- 1 tsp Tabasco sauce
- 2 tsp garlic powder
- 1.5 tsp cumin
- 1 tbsp kosher salt
- 1 tbsp black pepper
- 1 tsp paprika
- 1 tsp cayenne pepper
- 1 tsp dry mustard
- 2 tsp brown sugar
- 2 tsp Worcestershire sauce

Directions:

1. Mix all ingredients except ribs and barbecue sauce in a large bowl and rub it into the meat.

2. Wrap ribs in foil tightly and make sure no punctures have occurred.
3. Refrigerate the meat for at least one hour.
4. Put foil-wrapped ribs on a baking sheet and bake for 2 1/2 hours at 300 degrees Fahrenheit.
5. Baste the ribs with the barbecue sauce on both sides. Heat over a high flame on a grill for 10 minutes and serve.

Berry Treat Dessert

Ingredients:

- 4 cups of fresh mixed berries
- 1 cup whipping cream;
- 1 package of instant vanilla pudding
- 1/4 cup plus 2 tbsp of sugar
- 1 tsp vanilla
- 2 tbsp fresh lemon juice
- 24-36 purchased lady fingers

Directions:

1. Make pudding as directed on the package and chill.
2. Slice berries if necessary and add all berries, lemon juice and 1/4 cup sugar.
3. Whip the whipping cream, vanilla and 2 tbsp of sugar together until it forms soft peaks.
4. Put a layer of 7 lady fingers into a serving bowl.
5. Add a third of the berries and half the pudding.
6. Add more layers of lady fingers, berries and pudding.
7. Top with remaining lady fingers and add whipped cream and a berry garnish.

Spicy Pad Thai

Ingredients:

- 1-1/2 tsp olive oil
- 1/4 cup of ketchup
- 1 cup of coconut milk
- 2 tbsp evaporated can juice
- 2 tbsp of lime juice
- 3 tbsp soy sauce
- 12 ounces of Asian rice noodles
- 1 cup fresh bean sprouts
- 2 cups broccoli, chopped
- 2-3 garlic cloves, minced
- 1/3 cups cilantro
- a stalk of lemon grass, cut in thirds
- 4-6 scallions, thinly sliced
- 1 tsp dried red pepper flakes
- 1/3 cups peanuts

Directions:

1. Cook noodles until soft, then drain them.
2. Use a wok and heat the oil in it.
3. Sauté the garlic and add the lemon grass, scallions (the white part), and broccoli.
4. Steam until broccoli is completely tender.
5. Add noodles, greens of scallions and sauce.

6. Stir in red pepper flakes. Top with cilantro and peanuts.

Softened Sugar Cookies

Ingredients:

- 2 eggs
- 3-3/4 cup flour
- 1 cup butter or margarine (softened)
- 1.5 cups white sugar
- 1 tsp baking powder
- 1/2 tsp salt
- 2 tsp vanilla

Directions:

1. Mix sugar and butter in a bowl.
2. Beat in the eggs and vanilla and then add flour, baking powder, & salt.
3. Add mixture from Step 1 & stir thoroughly together.
4. Chill covered dough for 2 hours in the refrigerator.
5. Preheat oven at 400 degrees Fahrenheit.
6. On a floured surface, roll out dough and cut into shapes using cookie cutters.
7. If desired, decorate the cookies with sprinkles.
8. Bake for 6-8 minutes at 400 degrees or until the cookie edges are slightly brown.
9. Cool cookies on a wire rack.

Blueberry Banana Oatmeal

This is a great breakfast for someone with TMJ.

Ingredients:

- 1/2 cup oatmeal
- 1/2 cup sliced bananas
- 1 cup of water or milk
- 1/4 cup of frozen blueberries
- 2 tbsp walnuts, ground with a coffee grinder.

Directions:

1. Boil water and stir in oatmeal. Cook for about 3 1/2 minutes.
2. Stir in remaining ingredients.
3. Cook for an additional 1 1/2 minutes.
4. Let cool a bit and enjoy!

Luscious Potato Soup

This makes for a great supper!

Ingredients:

- 1/2 pound bacon, fried crispy
- 3 pounds red potatoes, diced
- 1/4 cup butter
- 1/4 cup flour
- 8 cups half and half
- 1 cup cheddar cheese
- 1 large package Velveeta cheese
- 1 tsp hot pepper sauce
- 1/2 cup freshly chopped parsley
- 1/2 fresh chives, chopped

Directions:

1. Boil potatoes in water until about three-fourths cooked.
2. Mix flour and melted butter to a smooth paste.
3. Slowly stir in half and half to the paste. Stir until smooth and thick.
4. Stir in melted Velveeta.
5. Drain the potatoes and mix them with the paste.
6. Add hot pepper sauce, garlic powder, and pepper.

7. Cook over low heat for about 30 minutes. Stir occasionally.
8. Top with bacon, parsley, chives, and shredded cheese.

Appetizers with Apples and Cheese

Ingredients:

- 3 cup peeled and sliced tart apples
- 1/2 tsp vanilla
- 1 tbsp butter
- 1/3 cup shredded cheddar cheese
- 1/2 tsp ground cinnamon
- 1/4 cup brown sugar, packed
- 1/4 cup raisins
- 1/8 tsp nutmeg
- Five 8-inch tortillas, warmed
- 10 tbsp whipped topping

Directions:

1. In a small pan, melt butter and dissolve brown sugar into butter.
2. Add cinnamon, apples, nutmeg, and raisins.
3. Cook over low to medium heat until apples are tenderized.
4. Take off the stove and stir in vanilla.
5. Pour 1/4 cup of mixture onto each tortilla. Fold over tortilla and wrap in foil wrap. Bake at 350 degrees for 10-12 minutes.
6. Sprinkle tortilla wraps with sugar and cinnamon. Top with whipped topping.

Eggnog Cookies

These are soft cookies for TMJ sufferers.

Ingredients:

- 1 egg
- 1/3 cup eggnog
- 2.5 cups flour
- 1/2 cup butter, unsalted
- 1 cup sugar
- 1/2 tsp salt
- 1 tsp vanilla
- 1/4 tsp rum extract
- 1/8 tsp nutmeg
- 1/2 cup baking soda

Directions:

1. Mix butter and sugar together and beat in the egg and extracts.
2. Add flour, salt, nutmeg, and baking soda alternating with eggnog so the whole thing is mixed together.
3. Drop tablespoonfuls of the mixture onto a baking sheet. Slightly flatten the cookie dough.
4. Bake at 375 degrees for 10-12 minutes.
5. For frosting, combine 2-3 tbsp softened butter, 3.5 cups confectioner's sugar, 1/4

cup eggnog, and 1/2 tsp vanilla. Sprinkle cinnamon or sugar on top.

Tortilla Turkey Soup

Ingredients:

- 1 cup turkey meat, diced
- 1 cup tomatoes, diced
- 1/2 cup canned black beans, rinsed & drained
- 1/2 cup onion, diced
- 1/2 cup frozen corn
- 1 tbsp vegetable oil
- 1-1/2 tbsp chili powder
- 1 tbsp tomato paste
- 4 cups chicken broth
- few sprigs cilantro
- salt to taste
- a package of tortilla strips
- shredded cheese and sour cream for garnish

Directions:

1. Sauté onions in vegetable oil for five minutes
2. Add tomato paste and chili powder. Stirring it so it doesn't scorch.
3. Add chicken broth, and cilantro. Bring to a boil.
4. Simmer until the broth has thickened by 1/3.

5. Remove cilantro sprigs.
6. Add turkey, tomatoes, salt, and beans. Heat thoroughly.
7. Place in bowls and garnish with sour cream, shredded cheese, and tortilla strips.

Turkey and French Onion Soup Casserole

Ingredients:

- 2 cups turkey, cooked & cubed
- 6 eggs
- 1 can condensed French onion soup
- 2 tbsp fresh thyme leaves, chopped
- 1 cup shredded cheese
- 2 cups milk
- 9 slices of crushed white bread, cubed or shredded

Directions:

1. Preheat oven to 350 degrees.
2. Beat together the eggs, soup, milk, 1/2 cup cheese and half of the thyme.
3. Add bread and turkey cubes, making sure the turkey and bread crumbs are coated.
4. Spray out a shallow baking dish using cooking spray.
5. Pour mixture into baking dish and sprinkle with remaining thyme and cheese.
6. Let stand for fifteen minutes, then bake for 45 minutes or until a knife comes out clean.

Tomato Soup and Croutons

Ingredients:

- 5 cups pulverized canned tomatoes including juice
- 1 onion, thinly sliced
- 2 tbsp butter
- 2 tbsp olive oil
- 3 garlic cloves, crushed
- 1/4 tsp celery seed
- 1 cup water
- 1/4 tsp oregano
- 1 tbsp sugar
- 2/3 cup heavy cream
- 1/4 crushed red pepper
- salt & pepper to taste
- 4 slices of bread diced about 3/4 inches by 3/4 inches

Directions:

1. Melt butter in a large saucepan and add olive oil.
2. Add onion and garlic and sauté.
3. Add tomatoes/juice, sugar, heavy cream, sugar, salt, pepper, crushed red pepper; oregano, and celery seed.
4. Bring soup to a boil, breaking up tomatoes so they are really crushed.

5. Reduce heat. Simmer for 10 minutes.
6. In a smaller skillet, cook rest of butter until it gets browned. Add olive oil and diced bread. Brown bread over about 6 minutes.
7. Puree the tomato soup in batches until perfectly smooth.
8. Add salt & pepper to taste.
9. Top with croutons & serve.

Stuffed Bell Peppers

Ingredients:

- 4 large yellow or red bell peppers
- 1 cup onions, chopped
- 1 stalk celery
- 1 medium can diced tomatoes with juice
- 1/2 cup oil-packed sun-dried tomatoes
- 1 tbsp olive oil
- 2 cloves minced garlic
- 1 can of kidney beans, drained
- 1/2 cup cooking wine
- 2 cup cooked brown rice
- 1 tbsp fresh basil, minced
- 2 tsp fresh oregano
- 1/2 cup dried currants
- 3/4 cup shredded Parmesan cheese
- 2 tsp jalapeno pepper, minced
- 1/8 tsp red pepper flakes
- Dash salt
- 1/4 tsp pepper
- 1 tsp sugar

Directions:

1. Preheat oven to 350 degrees. Oil an 8 X 10 inch baking pan.

2. Heat oil in large skillet. Add onions, garlic and celery. Sauté these ingredients.

3. Reduce heat. Add all other ingredients except peppers and Parmesan cheese.

4. Simmer for about 20 minutes.

5. Cut off and discard top part of bell pepper and remove interior seeds and ribs. Make sure pepper will stand up straight.

6. Spoon about 3/4 cup of sautéed ingredients into each pepper.

7. Cover peppers with tin foil and bake in pan for 30 minutes.

8. Uncover peppers, add parmesan cheese and bake for another 15 minutes.

Pumpkin Soup

Ingredients:

- 1 can pumpkin puree;
- 1 small onion, chopped;
- 1 green onion, top only;
- 1 cup vegetable broth;
- 3/4 cup water;
- 1/4 tsp nutmeg;
- 1/2 tsp cinnamon;
- 1 cup milk;
- 1/8 tsp black pepper.

Directions:

1. In a large saucepan, heat 1/4 cup water.
2. Add onion and cook for 3 minutes.
3. Add pumpkin, broth, spices, and rest of water.
4. Heat for 5 minutes and add milk until hot. Do not boil.
5. Top with green onion and black pepper.

Crème Brulee a la Oatmeal

Ingredients:

- 3 cup quick cook oatmeal
- 6 egg yolks
- 1 tsp vanilla
- 1/2 tsp salt
- 1/2 cup sugar
- 2 cups whipping cream
- 4 cups water
- 1/2 cup brown sugar
- 1/2 cup raisins

Directions:

1. Coat a slow cooker coated with oil or cooking spray. Preheat at high with lid closed.
2. Boil water and pour it into the slow cooker.
3. Add oatmeal, salt, and raisins. Close the lid.
4. In a bowl, mix egg yolks and granulated sugar. Set it aside.
5. Heat vanilla and whipping cream until just about to boil.
6. Whisk half cup of cream into eggs quickly. Blend the mixture well and spoon it over the cooked oatmeal.

7. Line the lid of the slow cooker with two paper towels and cover tightly. Cook on low for 3 hours.

Juicing for TMJ Disorder Patients

Because chewing hard things is difficult for TMJ sufferers and can exacerbate the symptoms, many sufferers turn to juicing for great nutrition and a chew-free diet. Juicing makes use of fresh ingredients that are juiced together using a blender or juice machine. Juicing is considered extremely friendly to those who have TMJ and can boost your immune system. It will break up veggies so the nutrition gets into your system easier. The fruits and veggies are great antioxidants that are anti-aging molecules. You can combine veggies and fruits for a sweet and great taste.

Here are some smoothies you can try in your blender or juicer:

Coffee Chocolate Smoothie. Take 1 cup of coffee, 1/2 cup of chocolate pudding, 2 scoops of vanilla ice cream, and 1/4 cup of ice. Blend in blender for a smooth coffee, chocolate taste.

Crème Orange Smoothie. Take 1 cup of milk, half cup of orange sherbet, and one package of Carnation instant breakfast mix (vanilla). Blend until smooth and creamy.

Apple Pie Smoothie. Take 2 cups of frozen ice cream or vanilla yogurt, 3/4 cup of unsweetened applesauce; 1/4 cup of apple juice; 1/2 tsp of cinnamon; 1/4 tsp of nutmeg; 1 cup of peeled and sliced apple. Blend first three ingredients for a few minutes and then add other ingredients, blending until the mixture is smooth.

Green Smoothie. Take one banana and a cup of frozen pineapple chunks. Add a few handfuls of fresh spinach or kale. Add about half cup of water and blend together for a tasty treat.

Energizing Smoothie. One mango cut in chunks, one banana, chopped, 1 cup of orange juice, 1 cup of nonfat vanilla yogurt. Blend together.

The idea behind eating for TMJ syndrome is to protect your bite by eating foods that aren't hard, crunchy or chewy and to get the nutrients known to protect those who have TMJ syndrome. If you have TMJ syndrome, choose some of the above recipes for the best in nutrients and that are soft enough to eat.

Brenda's story: *I lived with intractable TMJ pain for nearly five years before I came upon a recipe book especially designed for people with jaw problems. I had never associated my diet with my TMJ symptoms before I started choosing recipes from the book. What I enjoyed the most was that I could still eat delicious foods and the food didn't seem to make my jaw pain worse. I changed my entire diet and added a B complex vitamin for stress relief. After a few weeks, I could feel a change in the amount of pain I had and was finally free of the pain that had plagued me so long.*

Chapter 5: TMJ Relief with Exercise

TMJ disorder is a condition that is very amenable to exercise. By exercise, I don't mean running, jogging or swimming. These are exercises specific to TMJ disorder and are designed to strengthen the jaw muscles and help them learn to relax when necessary. Some say that exercise is the best possible option for those with TMJ disorder because it involves no medication and it can set you up with lasting habits that can help TMJ symptoms resolve completely.

The goal of exercise in the management of TMJ disorder is:

- To allow your jaw muscles to relax
- To strengthen the muscles around your TMJ
- To reduce the amount of popping and clicking of the TMJ

- To reduce pain associated with TMJ disorder
- To take the strain off of the joints, including the TMJ, around your jaw area.

Exercises for TMJ are often done twice daily for about five minutes at a time for each exercise. It is a good idea for you to try and do them first thing in the morning and just before going to bed. Just find a time you can do them quietly and without interruption. TMJ exercises are generally very safe for you to do but if you get too much soreness, you should discontinue the exercises and see a doctor or dentist.

One set of exercises begins with you having your mouth barely open. Put your right palm on the right side of your jaw. Move your jaw (mandible) toward your palm. Hold your hand in that position for about five seconds and replace the jaw into its proper position. Do this with the left side of your jaw as well. Repeat each exercise for a total of 5 times per side.

There are also isometric jaw exercises you can do. Place the palm of your hand on your chin and then jut out your chin as much as you can. Do this for five seconds and then re-peat the exercise for a total of 5 times.

There are neck stretching exercises that are helpful to TMJ disorder. These include rotating your neck to the right side, placing two fingers on your left jaw to push the neck further to the right. Hold for five seconds and repeat the same exercise on your left side. Repeat these exercises five times. Next, tilt your head upward so you are looking at the ceiling. Hold this position for about 5 seconds. You should feel a slight stretching sensation in your throat. Then drop your head so you are looking at the floor, feeling a slight stretching sensation in the back of the neck. Hold for five seconds and then repeat this position 5 times.

In the next exercise, you will touch your right ear to your right shoulder or approximate the two if your neck is too tight to actually touch your ear to your shoulder. Add some pressure using two fingers applied to the left temple. Hold the position for about 5 seconds. Repeat the exercise on the other side. You should do this exercise twice on each side.

The next exercise massages your TMJ joint muscles. Place three fingers on each temple. Massage the temples for a minimum of ten seconds. Be gentle with these muscles and don't put too much pressure on them. Repeat this massage technique for a total of 2-3 times. You can repeat this exercise as well by pushing and massaging the muscles in front of the ear (where the TMJ is located).

As for exercise you shouldn't do because it tends to make TMJ worse, avoid these things:

- Do not do much side to side chewing, which is the kind of movement you do when something is hard, chewy or crunchy. Even salads can be too crunchy for TMJ syndrome.
- Never chew gum. The constant chewing is bad for your jaw and TMJ.
- Don't open your mouth too wide as in biting a sandwich or yawning. Choose foods with smaller pieces.
- Attempt to keep your mouth slightly open and relaxed as possible. Do not set your teeth on edge as they will make things worse.
- Don't place your phone between your ear and shoulder.
- Don't support your jaw while sitting with the palm of your hand.

Hot compresses will sooth the jaw before or after exercises. The exercises alone will be able to take care of your TMJ pain if you practice them daily for several days or weeks, depending on how severe the problem is. Everyone has different degrees of TMJ pain and it may take longer if you have severe pain. Some people actually have pain relief after just one day's therapy. Be sure to be consistent in doing your TMJ exercises as skipping a day or two can throw off the TMJ completely so you will have to start all over again.

There are tracking improvement exercises that are supposed to eliminate popping, clicking and abnormal movement of the TMJ. You start by placing your tongue on the roof of the mouth. Put your index finger on your chin and the other at the area where the TMJ is located (in front of your ear). Open the jaw gradually and push it down and back toward your neck. Do this five times over for five sets a day each day. This helps stretch the muscles between your jawbone and your temporal bone.

You also need to strengthen the jaw. You start by sitting straight up on a bed or chair and release the tension from your body. Place a bent index finger inside your mouth, slightly opening the teeth. Keep your mouth open but remove your finger. Put your tongue on the roof of your mouth and use your index finger to put pressure on your jaw upward. Then apply pressure to the lower left side of the chin for two seconds and then repeat on the right side, keeping your jaw held tight in a neutral position. Repeat each exercise five times and then do five additional sets at various intervals throughout the day.

Jaw relaxation exercises are important, too. They reduce pain and keep the tension off the joints themselves. In one exercise, pain is reduced when you open your mouth slightly and then place two fingers on the middle of your bottom teeth. Press down to open the jaw to a comfortable position. Then release and repeat ten times, holding the position for 1-2 seconds at a time.

Next, put your tong onto the roof of your mouth and open your mouth widely while your tongue is still in the same position. Count a deep breath in for two seconds and a deep breath out for two seconds. Release the position and repeat this 10 times.

The next is an isotonic exercise. Put hour fist against the underside of your closed jaw. Try to open your jaw against the pressure being placed on it. Hold the tension for ten seconds. Repeat this exercise about 10 times in one day.

Next, press your fist against the right side of your jaw below the TMJ. Try to maintain steady pressure. This isometric pressure against the muscles of the TMJ and will allow these muscles to relax if you hold pressure for ten seconds, repeating it ten times. Do the same thing on the left side of your jaw.

Next, press the jaw on either side with one finger. Apply pressure evenly on both sides of the jaw. Open the jaw slowly, watching for clicking sounds. If the TMJ actually clicks, you must release the jaw and start over again, opening the jaw more slowly the next time. The alignment of the jaw must be perfect when you apply pressure to it with your fingers.

Once your jaw has become relaxed and is perfectly aligned, hold your chin between your thumb and index finger. Loosely and slowly, shake your chin back and forth so that your jaw releases itself and relaxes. Do this for about ten seconds and repeat as often as you need to during the day to feel less pain in your TMJ. Eventually, the jaw will learn to relax itself as it develops memory of being relaxed.

Exercise to the TMJ is perhaps the best way to get relief within just a few days. You can do them for a while and quit in order to see if the problem is resolved. TMJ syndrome, however, is usually long lasting so you need to expect to do these exercises for as long as it takes to get better and remain pain free.

Nathan's story: The last thing I expected when I saw my doctor for my TMJ pain was to have to do exercises. I kept thinking it was something they had to do surgery for. Instead, my doctor taught me a series of exercises that stretch and strengthen the jaw. I was supposed to do the exercises twice daily for a month and then report back to the doctor. The exercises themselves were easy to do. I found time to do them in the morning when I got up and in the evening before going to bed. Within two weeks, I began to feel better and when the month was up, I surprised my doctor by being pain free. I cut back on the exercises to once per day and I never again had TMJ symptoms as long as I kept up the exercises.

Chapter 6: Herbal and Home Remedies

There seems to be two schools of thought when it comes to TMJ disorder. We have already heard about the conventional school of thought that believes TMJ disorder is due to an abnormal dental bite and that it should best be treated with prescription medications and, if necessary, invasive surgery. The other school of thought recognizes that stress has a great deal to do with getting TMJ disorder and that the stress causes tension in the jaw muscles, throwing off the TMJ itself. The treatment, therefore, is to reduce stress through home remedies and possibly herbal remedies that decrease the underlying cause of TMJ disorder.

While you may be tempted to rush off to the dentist or doctor for invasive treatment, it is cheaper and just as effective in most cases to try home remedies to treat this disease and to get relief right away. Most home remedies are directed toward the pain, muscle tension and stress that together make TMJ disorder miserable. Let's look at some home remedies that you can do to quickly get that relief you need:

- **Massage.** Anytime you have muscle spasms causing severe pain in the TMJ, take three to four fingers and massage just in front of the ear on both sides opening and closing the jaw slowly as you do. It will take the spasm and tension out of the muscles, letting the joint loosen. The pain will go away as you do this for about five minutes at a time any time you have that spasmodic pain in the TMJ or just feel your jaw is too clenched.

- **Heat.** Heat is the best muscle relaxer you can get. Use a moist hot washcloth, a heating pad or a hot water bottle to the area overlying the TMJ or on the neck, jaw or shoulder muscles. This will loosen up tight muscles and secondarily ease the pain of TMJ disorder. Be careful you don't burn your skin in the process.

- **Ice packs.** Ice packs are great pain relievers. Many people alternate ice and heat so the pain can be relieved and the muscle spasm stopped. When you are really suffering, alternate heat and ice every 20 minutes. After you get relief, you should choose ice or heat (whichever feels the best) and stick with that until you get symptoms again.

- **Don't forget OTC pain relievers.** Acetaminophen, ibuprofen and naproxen work well for the relief of musculoskeletal pain. Try taking a reasonable dose of either of these and see how your pain is after a half hour. Switch to another pain reliever if others do not work.

- **Break old habits.** There are certain habits you may have that are exacerbating your condition, such as resting your head in the palm of your hand, putting the phone on your shoulder and tilting your head to one side so that you can get a grip on it and teeth clenching. For example, if you're a desk worker, make sure you sit up straight, raising your work surface higher so you don't stress your neck or jaw in the process of working on the computer or writing papers. Invest in a headset for your phone if you need both hands to talk on the phone or use speaker phone to keep your neck free. If you find yourself clenching your teeth when you're working say, on the computer, invest in a mouth guard or place a cork between your front teeth to keep your jaws relaxed and separated. It's good for your teeth to have it be this way, too.

- **Learn to relax.** Stress is a huge problem in patients with TMJ. If you can practice breathing techniques, progressive relaxation or yoga (mentioned earlier), you can learn how to relax the muscles of your whole body. Visualization techniques work well, too. You might have to take a ten minute break from work in order to find a quiet place for guided imagery or visualization. You can see yourself on a mountain meadow or possibly at the beach. Take slow deep breaths and hold this image for 5-10 minutes and then emerge relaxed with your jaw more relaxed. It's kind of like going on an emotional vacation for a few minutes.

- **Eat small pieces.** Cut or break your food into small pieces. Not only are these pieces easier to chew but they are easier to get in your mouth as well so you aren't hyperextending your jaw. When you yawn, try not to open your jaw much. Never bite into an apple, corn on the cob, caramels or other chewy candies. These can actually lock your jaw up in the open position, necessitating a visit to the emergency room to unlock it. Watch out for foods that are hard to chew, like bagels. They only make your bite off and can contribute to stress on the TMJ.

- **Don't chew gum.** This just adds extra pressure on your TMJ and will eventually wear away the structures of the joint.

- **Don't sleep on your stomach.** This puts extra pressure on one side of your face and can damage the TMJ over the years. Try using a cervical pillow that encourages you to sleep on your back when your jaw muscles are the most relaxed. Sleeping on your side isn't very good for your jaw, either.

- **Don't wear a heavy shoulder bag.** This just makes your shoulder muscles and neck muscles tense and puts extra tension on your TMJ. If you need to carry something heavy, do it with your hands or invest in a carrier that you can just pull along.

- **Practice exercises.** The exercises listed in the previous chapter can be done at home and work well to relieve the tension in the joints. Reread the chapter and practice these exercises at least twice a day for best relief.

- **Try Massage Therapy.** If you tell the massage therapist you're having TMJ problems and you'll get a focused massage involving your upper body and facial area. This will relax your TMJ and keep you pain-free for several days at least. Don't forget self-massage between visits to the massage therapist.

Homeopathic Treatments for TMJ

We've talked briefly about the role of homeopathy in treating TMJ syndrome. If you know a good homeopathic doctor, tell him or her about your symptoms and they will make a homeopathic remedy for you. Homeopathy involves diluting solutions of chemicals so they are tolerated and taken several times a day to resolve symptoms. Some homeopathic remedies for acute TMJ syndrome include a 30 times dilution four times daily. Chronic TMJ syndrome patients can get away with dilutions as little as 6 times potency, taken twice daily.

The remedies used include:

- **Arnica**. This is a great homeopathic remedy for deep, bruise-like pain. If your TMJ disorder was caused by an injury, arnica would be the remedy used.

- **Rhus Toxicodendron**. This is a remedy used for a stiffened jaw that is stiff in the morning, gets better during the day and then stiffens up at night. It is best taken warm for the fastest results.

- **Kali Phosphorica.** This reduces stress and pain caused by inflamed nerves.

- **Ignatia**. This is a remedy best used for those who clench their teeth and tighten their jaw because of stress. It is best used following an emotionally traumatic or grief reaction causing muscle tension in the face.

- **Magnesia Phosphorica.** This works best for those suffering from very tight muscles that wind up spasming at various times. It is best used while warm as it releases the tension in the muscles.

Herbal Remedies for TMJ

The herbal remedies/compounds used in TMJ disorder tend to be those that reduce stress, decrease inflammation of the TMJ joint and reduce pain. If you would like to use herbs to reduce your TMJ syndrome symptoms, seek out the services of a good herbalist who will direct you to the right herbal formula for your symptoms and will explain the right doses of each herbal ingredient.

There are herbs especially for bruxism that work as calming herbs, de-stressing your mind and body. When you are less stressed, you have decreased pain from TMJ symptoms. Some of the best herbs are as follows:

- **Blue Violet.** This has been used for thousands of years as an herbal remedy to relieve headaches and other pain. It can be made into a tea or used in capsule form. It contains methyl salicylate, which eases pain. It has anti-inflammatory power to decrease the inflammation in the TMJ, therefore decreasing pain.

- **Lobelia**. Lobelia is a powerful calmative and relaxant. You feel relaxed all over your body, including the neck, shoulder and facial area. It can make you sleepy if you don't take it with cayenne. Rarely can one be sensitive to it. It also relieves spasms of the muscles. Tinctures of lobelia can be rubbed onto affected spasmed areas or can be taken by dropfuls by mouth.

- **Kava**. This is a remedy that comes from the Pacific Southwest where it was used to relax people before ceremonies. In today's time, it is used as an anti-anxiety herbal medicine and relaxes the muscles.

- **St. John's Wort.** St. John's Wort is used by some as an antidepressant and by others as a way to relax the muscles and relieve spasm. By affecting the nervous system, it relaxes the mind and body so that people with TMJ have relief of nervous tension and pain.

- **Skullcap**. There are two kinds of skullcap, American skullcap and Chinese skullcap and it's the American version that works for TMJ disorder. Its use goes back more than 200 years and it is used as a mild relaxant to treat anxiety, muscle spasms and nervous tension. This is why it works so well for those who have TMJ disorder.

- **Catnip**. Catnip is used as an oil or herb parts are placed in capsules. It is an excellent remedy for anxiety, nervousness and sleep deprivation/insomnia. The chemical in the herb that causes the sedation is called nepetalactone, which, besides nervous tension, can relieve migraine headaches. It relaxes muscles so your TMJ disorder pain will be lessened. It relieves swelling caused by arthritis of the TMJ.

- **Thyme**. Thyme is an effective antispasmodic for tight muscles. It also acts on the joint itself with anti-inflammatory properties. It is often used in combination with other TMJ herbs.

- **Boswellia**. Boswellia has strong anti-inflammatory properties as well as anti-arthritic properties. If you have arthritis with clicking and popping of the joint, Boswellia may be the choice for you have arthritic changes in the TMJ itself. It has been tested and found functional against knee arthritis in at least one study.

- **Ginger**. Ginger has a great many properties, one of which is its anti-inflammatory properties against joint disease like TMJ. It is often used with herbs that work for relaxing the joints.

- **Nettle leaf**. This is the same plant people refer to as "stinging nettles". It has strong anti-inflammatory properties to relieve the symptoms of arthritis, such as is sometimes seen in TMJ disorder. It is often used with other anti-inflammatory herbs as well as herbs for relaxation of muscles. It also works for rheumatoid arthritis of the TMJ

- **Feverfew**. This is a great herbal remedy for TMJ disorder. It is good for soreness and pain and has strong anti-inflammatory properties. It is often used to treat headaches, muscle spasms and TMJ syndrome. This is a plant that belongs to the sunflower family and has been used for diseases like TMJ syndrome for many centuries.

While herbal remedies often have centuries of use in treating diseases like TMJ, they have the possibility of interacting with other herbs or with conventional medicines. This means you should contact either your doctor or your herbalist with a list of medications and herbal preparations you are taking so you don't get into any untoward reactions. Herbal remedies have the same pharmaceutical properties as some conventional drugs so you need to be aware of the possibility of doubling up on medications that shouldn't be doubled up or taken together.

Common sense remedies, simple exercises and herbal remedies can be used in almost all cases of temporomandibular joint disease so that you don't have to assume you are headed for invasive procedures to cure your disease. Much of what works for TMJ disorder is common sense. Anything that takes care of stress, muscle tension and inflammation can work to reduce the incidence of pain and stiffness of TMJ disorder—and this naturally includes herbal preparations.

Many herbal preparations for TMJ disorder are used together in combination capsules or in separate capsules. This is because you may need something for anxiety, something to relax the muscles and something to relieve pain or inflammation of the joint itself. Different herbs act on the different aspects of TMJ disorder and are needed to be taken together, similar to the way certain conventional medications are taken together.

Bethany's story: I developed TMJ disorder in my 30s. I think most of it was due to the stress of my job and to the stress of a divorce. I clearly needed something to relax the muscles of my face that were so tight they were causing my pain. I spoke to an herbalist who recommended that I try Kava and St. John's Wort. I could feel how the herbal remedies actually relaxed my mind and my muscles. Slowly, my pain began to dissipate and I felt normal again. I still take the herbal remedies because they have helped me so much to have a pain-free life again. I would recommend these herbs to anyone suffering from TMJ disorder.

Conclusion

Temporomandibular joint disease affects 20 million Americans, primarily women over men. It is a disease of tension in the joints located just in front of the ears and connecting the temporal bone to the mandible or jaw bone. Clenching of the teeth, bruxism or grinding of the teeth and an abnormal bite can cause the joint to receive excess pressure and begin to change the way the joint articulates. There can be structural changes such as bony prominences and abnormalities or dislocations of the soft meniscus that cushions that joint, which can cause pain and clicking of the joint.

The main symptoms of temporomandibular joint disease include pain in front of the ears where the TMJ is located, headache, migraines, stiffness of the jaw, a clicking or grinding sensation of the TMJ and an abnormal bite. Most people develop these symptoms between ages 20 and 40 years. Without treatment or management, the symptoms tend to get worse with age. They can be simply annoying symptoms or they can be so debilitating that you can't chew any hard food at all.

Much of what you do plays a role in managing TMJ disorder. There are recommendations to eat smaller bites, control the height of your yawn and to avoid holding the phone between the side of your head and your shoulder. Other recommendations include sleeping on your back instead of your stomach and wearing splints to keep the teeth from rubbing together, creating a bad bite.

Another part of the recommendations for TMJ disorder involve reducing stress and anxiety levels. Anytime you're under too much stress, you tend to clench your jaw. Too much of this and the muscles around the TMJ go into spasm and become inflamed, increasing the pain. The pain makes you clench your jaw even more so that you set up a vicious cycle of stress and muscle spasm. Breaking that cycle usually involves medications, exercises, meditation, or herbal remedies to loosen the muscle spasm through relief of mental stress.

For people who have dislocation of the spongy meniscus or severe arthritis to the affected joint, sometimes the doctor recommends arthroscopy, arthroscopic surgery or open joint surgery. These are, of course, treatments of last resort.

This guide offered you several different recipes so you could the idea of things you can eat that put little pressure on your teeth and your bite. By eating a diet of foods such as those listed in this guide, you put less tension on your jaw muscles and you still eat nutritiously. There are a few foods that are definitely off the list, such as peanuts and other crunchy or chewy foods. Fortunately, there are other things you can eat that will keep you full and pain-free when it comes to TMJ pain.

There are many different choices for pain relief when it comes to TMJ pain. Some are ultra-conservative and involve relaxation exercises and meditation. Others are more invasive and must be done by craniofacial specialists. Fortunately, most people can get by on conservative herbal remedies or exercises that can relieve the pain without doing anything invasive.

11040181R00058